Air Fryer Cookbook
Seafood Recipes

Top 50 Air Fryer Recipes with Low Salt, Low Fat and Less Oil.

The Healthier Way to Enjoy Deep-Fried Flavours

Ronda Williams

Table of Contents

Introduction

What is Air Frying?

First, a quick explanation of what air frying is and isn't. They don't fry food at all. They are more like a self-contained convection oven than a deep fat fryer. Most units have one or more heating elements, along with a fan or two to circulate the hot air. These appliances quickly heat and circulate the hot air around and through the food in the tray. This cooking method takes advantage of the heat and the drying effect of the air to cook foods quickly, leaving them crisp and browned on the outside but still moist inside. While the results can be similar to using a deep fryer, they are not identical.

What Are The Pros And Cons Of An Air Fryer?

While the enthusiasm about these products may be a bit overblown, there are some solid benefits to using an air fryer, as well as some major downsides.

Pros Of An Air Fryer

1. Healthier Meals

You do not need to use much (or any) oil in these appliances to get your food crispy and browned! Most users just spritz a little oil on the item and then proceed to the cooking cycle. The hot air takes advantage of the little bit of oil, and any excess oil just drains away from the food. This makes these devices ideal for making fresh and frozen fries, onion rings, mozzarella sticks, chicken wings, and nuggets. Unlike a traditional oven, air frying items are cooked faster and the excess oil doesn't soak into your food. So the claims that they use less oil and make healthier meals are true!

2. Quicker, More Efficient Cooking

Air fryers take just minutes to preheat, and most of the heat stays inside the appliance. Foods cook faster than in an oven or on a stovetop because this heat is not lost to the surrounding air. Even frozen foods are quickly cooked because the effect of the heat is intensified by the circulating air. These units are also more energy-efficient than an oven. Using a fryer will not heat your house in the summer, and the cost of the electricity used is just pennies. Since the cooking cycle is also shorter, you can see that using a fryer makes most cooking faster and more efficient than traditional appliances!

3. Versatility

You can use them to air fry, stir fry, reheat, bake, broil, roast, grill, steam, and even rotisserie in some models. Besides the fries and nuggets, you can make hot dogs and sausages, steak, chicken breasts or thighs, grilled sandwiches, stir-fried meats and veggies, roasted or steamed veggies, all kinds of fish and shrimp dishes, even cakes and desserts. If your unit is large enough, you can even bake a whole chicken or small turkey, or do a beef or pork roast. They are more than just a fryer!

4. Space-Saving

Most units are about the size of a coffee maker. Some models are small and super-compact, making them perfect for small kitchens, kitchenettes, dorm rooms, or RVs. An air fryer can replace an oven in a situation that lacks one and can be more useful than a toaster oven or steamer. If you use it frequently you will likely be happy to give it a home on your kitchen counter!

5. Easy To Use

Most fryers are designed to be easy to use. Just set the cooking temperature and time, put your food in the basket, and walk away. Of course, you will get better results if you shake your food once or twice during the cooking cycle, especially for things like fries, chips, wings, and nuggets. This ensures even browning and perfect results. Many air fryer enthusiasts have even taught their children to use them for making after school snacks or quick lunches!

Cons of an Air Fryer

1. Quality Issues

Air fryers are mostly made from plastic and inexpensive metal parts. They may or may not bear up after months or years of use. The heating elements, controls, and fans tend to go out eventually, and once they do your unit is useless. The metal cooking baskets and pans do not tend to last very long and often need to be replaced. Print on the dials or control panels can wear off. Even expensive units can have these issues, and some brands seem to have a lot of reported problems. These are not sturdy, long-lasting kitchen appliances overall.

2. Takes Up Space

Ok, I had "Space Saver" listed as a pro...how can it be a con as well? Easy! They do take up space, either on your counter or stored away in a cabinet. If you use it frequently this might not be a problem...but if you only drag it out to make the occasional batch of wings then the loss of space might not make it worth it to you. It depends on how and if you use it. Some units are fairly heavy as well, and might not be very easy to move around. They have the potential to be just another appliance you use a few times and then sell at a yard sale.

3. Not Ideal For Large Families

You will see some fryers advertised for "large families" but what does that mean? Most air fryers are best suited to making food for 1-4 people (depending on the capacity). There are very few that can handle making food for more than 4, and they often still require cooking in batches. For large families, a true convection air frying oven would probably be a better choice.

A medium-sized fryer with a capacity of 3.5 quarts can usually handle the main dish for two or a main and side dish for one. A large unit with a capacity of 5.8 quarts can handle the main dish like a whole chicken...which theoretically means enough to serve 4 people, as long as you cook the rest of the food in another appliance. So these are ideal for smaller families or single users, or a dorm or office snack maker.

4. Learning Curve

They ARE easy to use, but there is still a learning curve. Each unit has its peculiarities that you will have to figure out. They come with cooking guides and recipes, but those are more recommendations rather than firm instructions. It may take a few trials before you get the results that you want. Luckily the internet is filled with users who have shared their experiences, so finding tips is pretty easy.

5. Limitations

For all their versatility, air fryers have limitations as well. You are limited by the size and shape of the basket. Your frozen taquitos may not fit into some models, and you might be limited to a 6-inch pie pan in another. Food sometimes gets stuck to the cooking pans, meaning a more difficult clean-up for you. Even with accessories like elevated cooking racks and kabob skewers, you will still have to cook in batches or use another appliance if you are making food for multiple people. You also have to wait for the unit to cool off before cleaning and storing it away. For some people, these limitations might be too much to make an air fryer worth it.

Air Fryer Benefits

- An air fryer has many benefits to offer its customers.
- Low-fat meals
- Easy cleanup
- Uses hot-air circulation, the air fryer cooks your ingredients from all angles- with no oil needed.
- This ultimately produces healthier foods than most fryers and spares you from that unwanted aroma of fried foods in your home.
- To make sure you get the most out of your appliance, most fryers are accompanied by a recipe book to help you get started right away on your journey of fast, yet healthy meal preparations.

- Whether your favorite dish is french fries, muffins, chips, chicken tenders, or grilled vegetables, an air fryer can prepare it all.

Is an Air Fryer Useful?

At the tip of your fingers, you can have an appliance that specializes in making delicious, healthy meals that look and taste just like the ones made in oil fryers. The air fryer serves up many ways to be useful in your life.

Consider:

- Do you find yourself short on time to cook?
- Are you having a hard time letting go of those fatty foods, but still want to lose weight?
- Are you always seeking to get a bang for your buck?

If you answered yes to any of these questions, then an air fryer may be for you.

Why You Should Use An Air Fryer

An air fryer can pretty much do it all. And by all, we mean fry, grill, bake, and roast. Equipped with sturdy plastic and metal material, the air fryer has many great benefits to offer.

Air Fryers Can:

- Cook multiple dishes at once
- Cut back on fatty oils
- Prepare a meal within minutes
- While every appliance has its cons, the air fryer doesn't offer many.
- The fryer may be bulky in weight, but its dimensions are slimmer than most fryers. An air fryer can barely take up any counter space.
- If you need fast, healthy, convenient, and tasty, then once again, an air fryer may be for you.

Air Fryer- Healthier

The biggest quality the air fryer offers is healthier dishes

In comparison to other fryers, air fryers were designed to specifically function without fattening oils and to produce food with up to 80 percent less fat than food cooked with other fryers. The air fryer can help you lose the weight, you've been dying to get rid of. While it can be difficult to let go of your favorite fried foods, an air fryer will let you have your cake and eat it too. You can still have your fried dishes, but at the same time, still conserve those calories and saturated fat. The air fryer can also grill, bake, and roast foods as well. Offering you an all in one combination, the air fryer is the perfect appliance for anyone looking to switch to a healthier lifestyle.

Fast And Quick

- If you're on a tight schedule, you may want to use an air fryer.
- Within minutes you can have crunchy golden fries or crispy chicken tenders.
- This fryer is perfect for people who are constantly on the go and do not have much time to prepare meals.
- With most air fryers, french fries can be prepared within 12 minutes.
- That cuts the time you spend in the kitchen by a tremendous amount.

Features

1. Temperature And Timer

- Avoid the waiting time for your fryer to decide when it wants to heat up.
- With an air fryer, once you power it on, the fryer will instantly heat.
- When using the appliance cold, that is, right after it has been off for a while (since last use) all you have to do is add three minutes to your cooking time to allow for it to heat up properly.
- The appliance is equipped with adjustable temperature control that allows you to set the temperature that can be altered for each of your

meals.

- Most fryers can go up to 200-300 degrees.
- Because the fryer can cook food at record times, it comes with a timer that can be pre-set with no more than 30 minutes.
- You can even check on the progress of your foods without messing up the set time. Simply pull out the pan, and the fryer will cause heating. When you replace the pan, heating will resume.
- When your meal is prepared and your timer runs out, the fryer will alert you with its ready sound indicator. But just in-case you can't make it to the fryer when the timer goes, the fryer will automatically switch off to help prevent your ingredients from overcooking and burning.

2. Food Separator

Some air fryers are supplied with a food separator that enables you to prepare multiple meals at once. For example, if you wanted to prepare frozen chicken nuggets and french fries, you could use the separator to cook both ingredients at the same time, all the while avoiding the worry of the flavors mixing. An air fryer is perfect for quick and easy, lunch and dinner combinations. It is recommended to pair similar ingredients together when using the separator. This will allow both foods to share a similar temperature setting.

3. Air Filter

Some air fryers are built with an integrated air filter that eliminates those unwanted vapors and food odors from spreading around your house. No more smelling like your favorite fried foods, the air filter will diffuse that hot oil steam that floats and sticks. You can now enjoy your fresh kitchen smell before, during, and after using your air fryer.

4. Cleaning

- No need to fret after using an air fryer, it was designed for hassle-free cleaning.
- The parts of the fryer are constructed of non-stick material.
- This prevents any food from sticking to surfaces that ultimately make

it hard to clean.

- It is recommended to soak the parts of the appliances before cleaning.
- All parts such as the grill, pan, and basket are removable and dishwasher friendly.
- After your ingredients are cooked to perfection, you can simply place your parts in the dishwasher for a quick and easy clean.

Tips on Cleaning an Air Fryer:

- Use detergent that specializes in dissolving oil.
- For a maximum and quick cleaning, leave the pan to soak in water and detergent for a few minutes.
- Avoid using metal utensils when cleaning the appliance to prevent scuffs and scratches on the material.
- Always let the fryer cool off for about 30 minutes before you wash it.

5. Cost-effective

Are there any cost-effective air fryers? For all that they can do, air fryers can be worth the cost. It has been highly questionable if the benefits of an air fryer are worth the expense. When you weigh your pros and cons, the air fryer surely leads with its pros. There aren't many fryers on the market that can fry, bake, grill and roast; and also promise you healthier meals. An air fryer saves you time, and could potentially save you money. Whether the air fryer is cost-effective for your life, is ultimately up to you.

The air fryer is a highly recommendable appliance to anyone starting a new diet, parents with busy schedules, or individuals who are always on the go. Deciding whether the investment is worth it, is all up to the purchaser. By weighing the air fryer advantages and the unique differences the air fryer has, compared to other fryers, you should be able to decide whether the air fryer has a lot to bring to the table.

1. <u>Air Fryer Coconut Shrimp</u>

Prep Time: 30 mins

Cook Time: 15 mins

Total Time: 45 mins

Ingredient

- ½ cup all-purpose flour
- 1 ½ teaspoon ground black pepper
- 2 large eggs
- ⅔ cup unsweetened flaked coconut
- ⅓ cup panko bread crumbs
- 12 ounces uncooked medium shrimp, peeled and deveined
- cooking spray
- ½ teaspoon kosher salt, divided
- ¼ cup honey
- ¼ cup lime juice
- 1 serrano chile, thinly sliced
- 2 teaspoons chopped fresh cilantro

Instructions

- Stir together flour and pepper in a shallow dish. Lightly beat eggs in a second shallow dish. Stir together coconut and panko in a third shallow dish. Hold each shrimp by the tail, dredge in flour mixture, and shake off excess. Then dip floured shrimp in egg, and allow any excess to drip off. Finally, dredge in coconut mixture, pressing to adhere. Place on a plate. Coat shrimp well with cooking spray.
- Preheat air fryer to 400 degrees F (200 degrees C). Place 1/2 the shrimp in the air fryer and cook for about 3 minutes. Turn shrimp over and continue cooking until golden, about 3 minutes more. Season with 1/4 teaspoon salt. Repeat with remaining shrimp.
- Meanwhile, whisk together honey, lime juice, and serrano chile in a small bowl for the dip.

- Sprinkle fried shrimp with cilantro and serve with dip.

Nutrition Facts

Calories: 236; Protein 13.8g; Carbohydrates 27.6g; Fat 9.1g; Cholesterol 147.1mg; Sodium 316.4mg.

2. <u>Air-Fried Shrimp</u>

Prep Time: 5 mins

Cook Time: 10 mins

Total Time: 15 mins

Servings: 4

Ingredient

- 1 tablespoon butter, melted
- 1 teaspoon lemon juice
- ½ teaspoon garlic granules
- ⅛ teaspoon salt
- 1 pound large shrimp - peeled, deveined, and tails removed
- Perforated parchment paper
- ⅛ cup freshly grated parmesan cheese

Instructions

- Place melted butter in a medium bowl. Mix in lemon juice, garlic granules, and salt. Add shrimp and toss to coat.
- Line air fryer basket with perforated parchment paper. Place shrimp in the air fryer basket and sprinkle with Parmesan cheese.
- Cook shrimp in the air fryer at 400 degrees F (200 degrees C) until shrimp are bright pink on the outside and the meat is opaque for about 8 minutes.

Nutrition Facts

- Calories: 125; Protein 19.6g; Carbohydrates 0.5g; Fat 4.6g; Cholesterol 182.4mg; Sodium 329.7mg.

3. <u>Chef John's Salmon Cakes</u>

Prep Time: 15 mins

Cook Time: 10 mins

Additional Time: 30 mins

Total Time: 55 mins

Servings: 4

Ingredient

- 1 (14.75 ounces) can red salmon, skin, and bone removed, drained, and flaked
- 2 eggs
- ½ lemon, juiced
- 1 tablespoon chopped capers
- ½ teaspoon salt
- ½ teaspoon ground black pepper
- ½ teaspoon cayenne pepper
- 12 saltine crackers
- 1 tablespoon bread crumbs, or as needed
- 1 tablespoon butter
- 1 tablespoon olive oil

Instructions

- Stir salmon, eggs, lemon juice, capers, salt, black pepper, and cayenne pepper together in a bowl until well-combined.
- Crush saltine crackers with your hands into the salmon mixture and mix well. Wrap the bowl with plastic wrap and refrigerate, 30 minutes to overnight.
- Dust a plate with half the bread crumbs. Divide salmon mixture into 4 portions and shape into patties; place onto a prepared plate and sprinkle remaining bread crumbs atop the salmon patties.
- Melt butter and oil in a large skillet over medium heat. Cook patties in hot oil until cooked and heated through, about 5 minutes per side.

Nutrition Facts

- Calories: 305; Protein 30.9g; Carbohydrates 14.6g; Fat 14.6g; Cholesterol 174.2mg; Sodium 1019.9mg.

4. <u>Garlicky Appetizer Shrimp Scampi</u>

Prep Time: 15 mins

Cook Time: 6 mins

Total Time: 21 mins

Servings: 6

Ingredient

- 6 tablespoons unsalted butter, softened
- ¼ cup olive oil
- 1 tablespoon minced garlic
- 1 tablespoon minced shallots
- 2 tablespoons minced fresh chives
- Salt and freshly ground black pepper to taste
- ½ teaspoon paprika
- 2 pounds large shrimp - peeled and deveined

Instructions

- Preheat grill for high heat.
- In a large bowl, mix softened butter, olive oil, garlic, shallots, chives, salt, pepper, and paprika; add the shrimp, and toss to coat.
- Lightly oil grill grate. Cook the shrimp as close to the flame as possible for 2 to 3 minutes per side, or until opaque.

Nutrition Facts

- Calories: 303; Protein 25g; Carbohydrates 0.9g; Fat 21.8g; Cholesterol 261mg; Sodium 460.8mg.

5. <u>Grilled Fish Steaks</u>

Prep Time: 10 mins Cook Time: 10 mins Additional Time: 1 hr 10 mins

Total: 1 hr 30 mins

Servings: 2

Ingredient

- 1 clove garlic, minced
- 6 tablespoons olive oil
- 1 teaspoon dried basil
- 1 teaspoon salt
- 1 teaspoon ground black pepper
- 1 tablespoon fresh lemon juice
- 1 tablespoon chopped fresh parsley
- 2 (6 ounces) fillets of halibut

Instructions

- In a stainless steel or glass bowl, combine garlic, olive oil, basil, salt, pepper, lemon juice, and parsley.
- Place the halibut fillets in a shallow glass dish or a resealable plastic bag, and pour the marinade over the fish. Cover or seal and place in the refrigerator for 1 hour, turning occasionally.
- Preheat an outdoor grill for high heat and lightly oil grate. Set grate 4 inches from the heat.
- Remove halibut fillets from marinade and drain off the excess. Grill filets 5 minutes per side or until fish is done when easily flaked with a fork.

Nutrition Facts

- Calories: 554; Protein 36.3g; Carbohydrates 2.2g; Fat 43.7g; Cholesterol 62.5mg; Sodium 1259.3mg.

6. __Mussels Mariniere__

Prep Time: 35 mins

Cook Time: 15 mins

Total Time: 50 mins

Servings: 4

Ingredient

- 4 quarts mussels, cleaned and debearded
- 2 cloves garlic, minced
- 1 onion, chopped
- 6 tablespoons chopped fresh parsley
- 1 bay leaf
- ¼ teaspoon dried thyme
- 2 cups white wine
- 3 tablespoons butter, divided

Instructions

- Scrub mussels. Pull off beards, the tuft of fibers that attach each mussel to its shell, cutting them at the base with a paring knife. Discard those that do not close when you handle them and any with broken shells. Set aside.
- Combine onion, garlic, 4 tablespoons parsley, bay leaf, thyme, wine, and 2 tablespoons butter in a large pot. Bring to boil. Lower heat, and cook for 2 minutes. Add mussels, and cover. Cook just until shells open, 3 to 4 minutes. Do not overcook. Remove mussels from the sauce, and place in bowls.
- Strain liquid, and return to pot. Add remaining butter and parsley. Heat until butter melts. Pour over mussels.

Nutrition Facts

- Calories: 298; Protein 18.6g; Carbohydrates 10.3g; Fat 10.1g; Cholesterol 69.6mg; Sodium 329.6mg.

7. Chef John's Baked Lemon Pepper Salmon

Prep Time: 10 mins Cook Time: 15 mins Additional Time: 30 mins Total Time: 55 mins Servings: 2

Ingredient

- 2 tablespoons lemon juice
- 1 tablespoon ground black pepper
- 1 ½ tablespoons mayonnaise
- 1 tablespoon yellow miso paste
- 2 teaspoons dijon mustard
- 1 pinch cayenne pepper, or to taste
- 2 (8 ounces) center-cut salmon fillets, boned, skin on
- Sea salt to taste

Instructions

- Whisk together lemon juice and black pepper in a small bowl. Add mayonnaise, miso paste, Dijon mustard, and cayenne pepper to lemon-pepper mixture; whisk together.
- Spread the lemon-pepper mixture over salmon fillets. Reserve about a tablespoon for later use.
- Cover salmon with plastic wrap and refrigerate for 30 minutes.
- Preheat oven to 450 degrees F (230 degrees C). Line a baking sheet with parchment paper or a silicone baking mat.
- Place fillets on the prepared baking sheet. Spread the remaining lemon-pepper mixture on fillets without letting it pool around the base. Sprinkle with a pinch more black pepper and a generous amount of sea salt.
- Bake in the preheated oven until the fish flakes easily with a fork, 10 to 15 minutes.

Nutrition Facts

- Calories: 488; Protein 49.5g; Carbohydrates 7.1g; Fat 28.1g; Cholesterol 156.6mg; Sodium 784.3mg.

8. <u>Rockin' Oysters Rockefeller</u>

Prep Time: 30 mins

Cook Time: 30 mins

Total Time: 1 hr

Servings: 16

Ingredient

- 48 fresh, unopened oysters
- 1 ½ cups beer
- 2 cloves garlic
- seasoned salt to taste
- 7 black peppercorns
- ½ cup butter
- 1 onion, chopped
- 1 clove garlic, crushed
- 1 (10 ounces) package frozen chopped spinach, thawed and drained
- 8 ounces Monterey Jack cheese, shredded
- 8 ounces fontina cheese, shredded
- 8 ounces mozzarella cheese, shredded
- ½ cup milk
- 2 teaspoons salt, or to taste
- 1 teaspoon ground black pepper
- 2 tablespoons fine bread crumbs

Instructions

- Clean oysters, and place them in a large stockpot. Pour in beer and enough water to cover oysters; add 2 cloves garlic, seasoned salt, and peppercorns. Bring to a boil. Remove from heat, drain, and cool.
- Once oysters are cooled, break off and discard the top shell. Arrange the oysters on a baking sheet. Preheat oven to 425 degrees F (220 degrees C.)
- Melt butter in a saucepan over medium heat. Cook onion and garlic in butter until soft. Reduce heat to low, and stir in spinach, Monterey

Jack, fontina, and mozzarella. Cook until cheese melts, stirring frequently. Stir in the milk, and season with salt and pepper. Spoon sauce over each oyster, just filling the shell. Sprinkle with bread crumbs.

- Bake until golden and bubbly, approximately 8 to 10 minutes.

Nutrition Facts

- Calories: 248; Protein 16.4g; Carbohydrates 5.3g; Fat 17.4g; Cholesterol 65.7mg; Sodium 652.2mg.

9. <u>Sesame Seared Tuna</u>

Prep Time: 10 mins

Cook Time: 10 mins

Total Time: 20 mins

Servings: 4

Ingredient

- ¼ Cup soy sauce
- 1 tablespoon mirin (japanese sweet wine)
- 1 tablespoon honey
- 2 tablespoons sesame oil
- 1 tablespoon rice wine vinegar
- 4 (6 ounces) tuna steaks
- ½ cup sesame seeds
- Wasabi paste
- 1 tablespoon olive oil

Instructions

- In a small bowl, stir together the soy sauce, mirin, honey, and sesame oil. Divide into two equal parts. Stir the rice vinegar into one part and set aside as a dipping sauce.
- Spread the sesame seeds out on a plate. Coat the tuna steaks with the remaining soy sauce mixture, then press into the sesame seeds to coat.
- Heat olive oil in a cast-iron skillet over high heat until very hot. Place steaks in the pan, and sear for about 30 seconds on each side. Serve with the dipping sauce and wasabi paste.

Nutrition Facts

Calories: 422; Protein 44.1g; Carbohydrates 13.2g; Fat 20.7g; Cholesterol 77.2mg; Sodium 1045.5mg.

10. **<u>Dinah's Baked Scallops</u>**

Prep Time: 20 mins

Cook Time: 15 mins

Total Time: 35 mins

Servings: 4

Ingredient

- 20 buttery round crackers, crushed
- black pepper to taste
- 1 teaspoon garlic powder
- 1 pound sea scallops, rinsed and drained
- ½ cup butter, melted
- ¼ cup dry white wine
- ½ lemon, juiced
- 1 tablespoon chopped fresh parsley, for garnish

Instructions

- Preheat oven to 350 degrees F (175 degrees C). Lightly grease an 8x8 inch baking dish.
- Combine crushed crackers, black pepper, and garlic powder in a small bowl. Press scallops into the mixture so that they are evenly coated, and place them in the greased baking dish.
- In a separate bowl, mix melted butter, wine, and lemon juice; drizzle mixture over scallops.
- Bake in the preheated oven until scallops are lightly browned, about 15 minutes. Garnish with chopped parsley.

Nutrition Facts

- Calories: 431; Protein 19.7g; Carbohydrates 15.3g; Fat 31.5g; Cholesterol 96.5mg; Sodium 530.1mg.

11.   Easy-Bake Fish

Prep Time: 15 mins

Cook Time: 20 mins

Total Time: 35 mins

Servings: 4

Ingredient

- 3 tablespoons honey
- 3 tablespoons Dijon mustard
- 1 teaspoon lemon juice
- 4 (6 ounces) salmon steaks
- ½ teaspoon pepper

Instructions

- Preheat oven to 325 degrees F (165 degrees C).
- In a small bowl, mix honey, mustard, and lemon juice. Spread the mixture over the salmon steaks. Season with pepper. Arrange in a medium baking dish.
- Bake 20 minutes in the preheated oven, or until fish easily flakes with a fork.

Nutrition Facts

- Calories: 368; Protein 33.5g; Carbohydrates 15.6g; Fat 18.2g; Cholesterol 99.1mg; Sodium 381.1mg.

12.   Seared Scallops With Jalapeno Vinaigrette

Prep Time: 5 mins

Cook Time: 10 mins

Total Time: 15 mins

Servings: 4

Ingredient

- 1 large jalapeno pepper, seeded and membranes removed
- ¼ cup rice vinegar
- ¼ cup olive oil
- ¼ teaspoon dijon mustard
- Salt and freshly ground black pepper to taste
- 1 tablespoon vegetable oil
- 12 large fresh sea scallops
- 1 pinch sea salt
- 1 pinch cayenne pepper
- 2 oranges, peeled and cut in between sections as segments

Instructions

- Place jalapeno, rice vinegar, olive oil, and Dijon mustard in a blender. Puree on high until mixture is completely liquefied, 1 to 2 minutes. Season with salt and black pepper to taste.
- Season scallops with sea salt and cayenne pepper. Heat vegetable oil in a skillet over high heat. Place scallops in skillet and cook until browned, 2 to 3 minutes per side. Transfer to a plate. Garnish scallops with orange segments and drizzle jalapeno vinaigrette over the top.

Nutrition Facts

- Calories: 307; Protein 30.1g; Carbohydrates 5.9g; Fat 18g; Cholesterol 72.4mg; Sodium 472mg.

13. Hudson's Baked Tilapia With Dill Sauce

Prep Time: 10 mins Cook Time: 20 mins Total Time: 30 mins

Servings: 4

Ingredient

- 4 (4 ounce) fillets tilapia
- Salt and pepper to taste
- 1 tablespoon cajun seasoning, or to taste
- 1 lemon, thinly sliced
- ¼ cup mayonnaise
- ½ cup sour cream
- ⅛ teaspoon garlic powder
- 1 teaspoon fresh lemon juice
- 2 tablespoons chopped fresh dill

Instructions

- Preheat the oven to 350 degrees F (175 degrees C). Lightly grease a 9x13 inch baking dish.
- Season the tilapia fillets with salt, pepper, and Cajun seasoning on both sides. Arrange the seasoned fillets in a single layer in the baking dish. Place a layer of lemon slices over the fish fillets. I usually use about 2 slices on each piece so that it covers most of the surface of the fish.
- Bake uncovered for 15 to 20 minutes in the preheated oven, or until fish flakes easily with a fork.
- While the fish is baking, mix the mayonnaise, sour cream, garlic powder, lemon juice, and dill in a small bowl. Serve with tilapia.

Nutrition Facts

- Calories: 284; Protein 24.5g; Carbohydrates 5.7g; Fat 18.6g; Cholesterol 58.9mg; Sodium 500.5mg.

14.   Angy Lemon-Garlic Shrimp

Prep Time: 10 mins

Cook Time: 10 mins

Total Time: 20 mins

Servings: 4

Ingredient

- 16 large shrimp - peeled, deveined, and tails on, or more to taste
- 3 large cloves garlic, smashed, or more to taste
- 1 teaspoon crushed red pepper, or to taste
- 2 teaspoons seafood seasoning (such as old bay®), or to taste
- Salt and ground black pepper to taste
- 2 tablespoons lemon juice
- 3 tablespoons chopped fresh parsley
- 3 teaspoons lemon zest

Instructions

- Heat a large skillet over medium-low heat until warm, about 3 minutes. Add shrimp, garlic, and crushed red pepper all at once and stir together. Add seafood seasoning, salt, and black pepper. Mix everything.
- Cook over medium heat until shrimp are fully cooked, 3 to 5 minutes. Pour lemon juice into skillet and stir again. Reduce heat to low; add parsley and lemon zest. Transfer only shrimp to a serving platter.

Nutrition Facts

- Calories: 76; Protein 14.2g; Carbohydrates 2.4g; Fat 0.9g; Cholesterol 127.7mg; Sodium 460.3mg.

15. **Parmesan-Crusted Shrimp Scampi With Pasta**

Prep Time: 25 mins

Cook Time: 20 mins

Total Time: 45 mins

Servings: 6

Ingredient

- 2 cups angel hair pasta
- ½ cup butter, divided
- 4 cloves garlic, minced
- 1 pound uncooked medium shrimp, peeled and deveined
- ½ cup white cooking wine
- 1 lemon, juiced
- 1 teaspoon red pepper flakes
- ¾ cup seasoned bread crumbs
- ¾ cup freshly grated Parmesan cheese, divided
- 2 tablespoons finely chopped fresh parsley

Instructions

- Bring a large pot of lightly salted water to a boil. Cook angel hair pasta in the boiling water, stirring occasionally, until tender yet firm to the bite, 4 to 5 minutes. Drain and set aside.
- Set an oven rack about 6 inches from the heat source and preheat the oven's broiler.
- Heat 1/4 cup butter over medium heat in a large, deep skillet. Add garlic; cook and stir until fragrant. Add shrimp, white wine, and lemon juice; continue to cook and stir until shrimp is bright pink on the outside and the meat is opaque about 5 minutes. Stir in red pepper flakes until well combined. Remove from heat and set aside.
- Place remaining 1/4 cup butter, bread crumbs, 1/2 the Parmesan cheese, and parsley in a bowl. Stir until well combined. Set aside.

- Place cooked pasta into shrimp scampi mixture; toss until fully coated in sauce. Add remaining Parmesan cheese and toss well. Top with bread crumb mixture.
- Broil in the preheated oven until golden brown, 3 to 4 minutes. Serve immediately.

Nutrition Facts

- Calories: 419; Protein 22.6g; Carbohydrates 33.4g; Fat 20.8g; Cholesterol 164.7mg; Sodium 731.6mg.

16. Chef John's Fresh Salmon Cakes

Prep Time: 20 mins

Cook Time: 15 mins

Additional Time: 1 hr

Total Time: 1 hr 35 mins

Servings: 4

Ingredient

- 1 tablespoon extra-virgin olive oil
- ¼ cup minced onion
- 2 tablespoons minced red bell pepper
- 2 tablespoons minced celery
- Salt and pepper to taste
- 1 tablespoon capers
- 1 ¼ pound fresh wild salmon, coarsely chopped
- ¼ cup mayonnaise
- ¼ cup panko bread crumbs
- 2 cloves garlic, minced
- 1 teaspoon dijon mustard
- 1 pinch cayenne pepper
- 1 pinch seafood seasoning (such as old bay®)
- 1 tablespoon panko bread crumbs, or to taste
- 2 tablespoons olive oil, or as needed

Instructions

- Heat extra virgin olive oil in a skillet over medium heat. Cook and stir onion, red pepper, celery, and a pinch of salt in hot oil until onion is soft and translucent about 5 minutes. Add capers; cook and stir until fragrant, about 2 minutes. Remove from heat and cool to room temperature.
- Stir salmon, onion mixture, mayonnaise, 1/4 cup bread crumbs, garlic, mustard, cayenne, seafood seasoning, salt, and ground black

pepper together in a bowl until well-mixed. Cover the bowl with plastic wrap and refrigerate until firmed and chilled, 1 to 2 hours.

- Form salmon mixture into four 1-inch thick patties; sprinkle remaining panko bread crumbs over each patty.
- Heat olive oil in a skillet over medium heat. Cook patties in hot oil until golden and cooked through, 3 to 4 minutes per side.

Nutrition Facts

- Calories: 460; Protein 31.6g; Carbohydrates 8.5g; Fat 33.5g; Cholesterol 101.6mg; Sodium 337.3mg.

17. **<u>Best Tuna Casserole</u>**

Prep Time: 15 mins

Cook Time: 20 mins

Total Time: 35 mins

Servings: 6

Ingredient

- 1 (12 ounces) package egg noodles
- ¼ cup chopped onion
- 2 cups shredded Cheddar cheese
- 1 cup frozen green peas
- 2 (5 ounce) cans tuna, drained
- 2 (10.75 ounces) cans condensed cream of mushroom soup
- ½ (4.5 ounces) can sliced mushrooms
- 1 cup crushed potato chips

Instructions

- Bring a large pot of lightly salted water to a boil. Cook pasta in boiling water for 8 to 10 minutes, or until al dente; drain.
- Preheat oven to 425 degrees F (220 degrees C).
- In a large bowl, thoroughly mix noodles, onion, 1 cup cheese, peas, tuna, soup, and mushrooms. Transfer to a 9x13 inch baking dish, and top with potato chip crumbs and remaining 1 cup cheese.
- Bake for 15 to 20 minutes in the preheated oven, or until cheese is bubbly.

Nutrition Facts

- Calories: 595; Protein 32.1g; Carbohydrates 58.1g; Fat 26.1g; Cholesterol 99.2mg; Sodium 1061.1mg

18.   Good New Orleans Creole Gumbo

Prep Time: 1 hr

Cook Time: 2 hrs 40 mins

Total Time: 3 hrs 40 mins

Servings: 20

Ingredient

- 1 cup all-purpose flour
- ¾ cup bacon drippings
- 1 cup coarsely chopped celery
- 1 large onion, coarsely chopped
- 1 large green bell pepper, coarsely chopped
- 2 cloves garlic, minced
- 1 pound andouille sausage, sliced
- 3 quarts water
- 6 cubes beef bouillon
- 1 tablespoon white sugar
- Salt to taste
- 2 tablespoons hot pepper sauce (such as tabasco®), or to taste
- ½ teaspoon cajun seasoning blend (such as tony chachere's), or to taste
- 4 bay leaves
- ½ teaspoon dried thyme leaves
- 1 (14.5 ounces) can stewed tomatoes
- 1 (6 ounces) can tomato sauce
- 4 teaspoons file powder, divided
- 2 tablespoons bacon drippings
- 2 (10 ounces) packages frozen cut okra, thawed
- 2 tablespoons distilled white vinegar
- 1 pound lump crabmeat
- 3 pounds uncooked medium shrimp, peeled and deveined
- 2 tablespoons worcestershire sauce

Instructions

- Make a roux by whisking the flour and 3/4 cup bacon drippings together in a large, heavy saucepan over medium-low heat to form a smooth mixture. Cook the roux, whisking constantly until it turns a rich mahogany brown color. This can take 20 to 30 minutes; watch heat carefully and whisk constantly or roux will burn. Remove from heat; continue whisking until the mixture stops cooking.
- Place the celery, onion, green bell pepper, and garlic into the work bowl of a food processor, and pulse until the vegetables are very finely chopped. Stir the vegetables into the roux, and mix in the sausage. Bring the mixture to a simmer over medium-low heat, and cook until vegetables are tender, 10 to 15 minutes. Remove from heat, and set aside.
- Bring the water and beef bouillon cubes to a boil in a large Dutch oven or soup pot. Stir until the bouillon cubes dissolve, and whisk the roux mixture into the boiling water. Reduce heat to a simmer, and mix in the sugar, salt, hot pepper sauce, Cajun seasoning, bay leaves, thyme, stewed tomatoes, and tomato sauce. Simmer the soup over low heat for 1 hour; mix in 2 teaspoons of file gumbo powder at the 45-minute mark.
- Meanwhile, melt 2 tablespoons of bacon drippings in a skillet, and cook the okra with vinegar over medium heat for 15 minutes; remove okra with a slotted spoon, and stir into the simmering gumbo. Mix in crabmeat, shrimp, and Worcestershire sauce, and simmer until flavors have blended, 45 more minutes. Just before serving, stir in 2 more teaspoons of file gumbo powder.

Nutrition Facts

- Calories: 283; Protein 20.9g; Carbohydrates 12.1g; Fat 16.6g; Cholesterol 142.6mg; Sodium 853.1mg.

19. <u>**Shrimp Scampi With Pasta**</u>

Prep Time: 20 mins

Cook Time: 20 mins

Total Time: 40 mins

Servings: 6

Ingredient

- 1 (16 ounces) package linguine pasta
- 2 tablespoons butter
- 2 tablespoons extra-virgin olive oil
- 2 shallots, finely diced
- 2 cloves garlic, minced
- 1 pinch red pepper flakes (optional)
- 1 pound shrimp, peeled and deveined
- 1 pinch kosher salt and freshly ground pepper
- ½ cup dry white wine
- 1 lemon, juiced
- 2 tablespoons butter
- 2 tablespoons extra-virgin olive oil
- ¼ cup finely chopped fresh parsley leaves
- 1 teaspoon extra-virgin olive oil, or to taste

Instruction

- Bring a large pot of salted water to a boil; cook linguine in boiling water until nearly tender, 6 to 8 minutes. Drain.
- Melt 2 tablespoons butter with 2 tablespoons olive oil in a large skillet over medium heat. Cook and stir shallots, garlic, and red pepper flakes in the hot butter and oil until shallots are translucent, 3 to 4 minutes. Season shrimp with kosher salt and black pepper; add to the skillet and cook until pink, stirring occasionally, 2 to 3 minutes. Remove shrimp from skillet and keep warm.
- Pour white wine and lemon juice into skillet and bring to a boil while scraping the browned bits of food off of the bottom of the skillet with

37

a wooden spoon. Melt 2 tablespoons butter in a skillet, stir 2 tablespoons olive oil into butter mixture, and bring to a simmer. Toss linguine, shrimp, and parsley in the butter mixture until coated; season with salt and black pepper. Drizzle with 1 teaspoon olive oil to serve.

Nutrition Facts

- Calories: 511; Protein 21.9g; Carbohydrates 57.5g; Fat 19.4g; Cholesterol 135.4mg; Sodium 260mg.

20. Easy Garlic-Lemon Scallops

Prep Time: 10 mins

Cook Time: 10 mins

Total Time: 20 mins

Servings: 6

Ingredient

- ¾ cup butter
- 3 tablespoons minced garlic
- 2 pounds large sea scallops
- 1 teaspoon salt
- ⅛ teaspoon pepper
- 2 tablespoons fresh lemon juice

Instructions

- Melt butter in a large skillet over medium-high heat. Stir in garlic, and cook for a few seconds until fragrant. Add scallops, and cook for several minutes on one side, then turn over, and continue cooking until firm and opaque.
- Remove scallops to a platter, then whisk salt, pepper, and lemon juice into butter. Pour sauce over scallops to serve.

Nutrition Facts

- Calories: 408; Protein 38.5g; Carbohydrates 8.9g; Fat 24.4g; Cholesterol 152.4mg; Sodium 987.9mg.

21.   **Perfect Ten Baked Cod**

Prep Time: 10 mins

Cook Time: 25 mins

Total Time: 35 mins

Servings: 4

Ingredient

- 2 tablespoons butter
- ½ sleeve buttery round crackers (such as Ritz®), crushed
- 2 tablespoons butter
- 1 pound thick-cut cod loin
- ½ lemon, juiced
- ¼ cup dry white wine
- 1 tablespoon chopped fresh parsley
- 1 tablespoon chopped green onion
- 1 lemon, cut into wedges

Instructions

- Preheat oven to 400 degrees F (200 degrees C).
- Place 2 tablespoons butter in a microwave-safe bowl; melt in the microwave on high, about 30 seconds. Stir buttery round crackers into melted butter.
- Place remaining 2 tablespoons butter in a 7x11-inch baking dish. Melt in the preheated oven, 1 to 3 minutes. Remove dish from oven.
- Coat both sides of cod in melted butter in the baking dish.
- Bake cod in the preheated oven for 10 minutes. Remove from oven; top with lemon juice, wine, and cracker mixture. Place back in the oven and bake until fish is opaque and flakes easily with a fork, about 10 more minutes.
- Garnish baked cod with parsley and green onion. Serve with lemon wedges.

Nutrition Facts

- Calories: 280; Protein 20.9g; Carbohydrates 9.3g; Fat 16.1g; Cholesterol 71.5mg; Sodium 282.3mg.

22. Marinated Tuna Steak

Prep Time: 10 mins

Cook Time: 11 mins

Additional Time: 30 mins

Total Time: 51 mins

Servings: 4

Ingredient

- ¼ cup orange juice
- ¼ cup soy sauce
- 2 tablespoons olive oil
- 1 tablespoon lemon juice
- 2 tablespoons chopped fresh parsley
- 1 clove garlic, minced
- ½ teaspoon chopped fresh oregano
- ½ teaspoon ground black pepper
- 4 (4 ounces) tuna steaks

Instructions

- In a large non-reactive dish, mix the orange juice, soy sauce, olive oil, lemon juice, parsley, garlic, oregano, and pepper. Place the tuna steaks in the marinade and turn to coat. Cover, and refrigerate for at least 30 minutes.
- Preheat grill for high heat.
- Lightly oil grill grate. Cook the tuna steaks for 5 to 6 minutes, then turn and baste with the marinade. Cook for an additional 5 minutes, or to the desired doneness. Discard any remaining marinade.

Nutrition Facts

- Calories: 200; Protein 27.4g; Carbohydrates 3.7g; Fat 7.9g; Cholesterol 50.6mg; Sodium 944.6mg.

23. Seared Ahi Tuna Steaks

Prep Time: 5 mins

Cook Time: 12 mins

Total Time: 17 mins

Servings: 2

Ingredient

- 2 (5 ounces) ahi tuna steaks
- 1 teaspoon kosher salt
- ¼ teaspoon cayenne pepper
- ½ tablespoon butter
- 2 tablespoons olive oil
- 1 teaspoon whole peppercorns

Instructions

Season the tuna steaks with salt and cayenne pepper.

Melt the butter with the olive oil in a skillet over medium-high heat. Cook the peppercorns in the mixture until they soften and pop about 5 minutes. Gently place the seasoned tuna in the skillet and cook to desired doneness, 1 1/2 minutes per side for rare.

Nutrition Facts

- Calories: 301; protein 33.3g; carbohydrates 0.7g; fat 17.8g; cholesterol 71.4mg; sodium 1033.6mg.

24. Easy Paella

Prep Time: 30 mins

Cook Time: 30 mins

Total Time: 1 hr

Servings: 8

Ingredient

- 2 tablespoons olive oil
- 1 tablespoon paprika
- 2 teaspoons dried oregano
- Salt and black pepper to taste
- 2 pounds skinless, boneless chicken breasts, cut into 2-inch pieces
- 2 tablespoons olive oil, divided
- 3 cloves garlic, crushed
- 1 teaspoon crushed red pepper flakes
- 2 cups uncooked short-grain white rice
- 1 pinch saffron threads
- 1 bay leaf
- ½ bunch italian flat-leaf parsley, chopped
- 1-quart chicken stock
- 2 lemons, zested
- 2 tablespoons olive oil
- 1 spanish onion, chopped
- 1 red bell pepper, coarsely chopped
- 1 pound chorizo sausage, casings removed and crumbled
- 1 pound shrimp, peeled and deveined

Instructions

- In a medium bowl, mix 2 tablespoons of olive oil, paprika, oregano, and salt and pepper. Stir in chicken pieces to coat. Cover, and refrigerate.
- Heat 2 tablespoons olive oil in a large skillet or paella pan over medium heat. Stir in garlic, red pepper flakes, and rice. Cook, stirring,

44

to coat the rice with oil, about 3 minutes. Stir in saffron threads, bay leaf, parsley, chicken stock, and lemon zest. Bring to a boil, cover, and reduce heat to medium-low. Simmer 20 minutes.

- Meanwhile, heat 2 tablespoons olive oil in a separate skillet over medium heat. Stir in marinated chicken and onion; cook 5 minutes. Stir in bell pepper and sausage; cook 5 minutes. Stir in shrimp; cook, turning the shrimp until both sides are pink.
- Spread rice mixture onto a serving tray. Top with meat and seafood mixture.

Nutrition Facts

- Calories: 736; Protein 55.7g; Carbohydrates 45.7g; Fat 35.1g; Cholesterol 202.5mg; Sodium 1204.2mg.

25. <u>Simple Garlic Shrimp</u>

Prep Time: 15 mins

Cook Time: 10 mins

Total Time: 25 mins

Servings: 4

Ingredient

- 1 ½ tablespoon olive oil
- 1 pound shrimp, peeled and deveined
- Salt to taste
- 6 cloves garlic, finely minced
- ¼ teaspoon red pepper flakes
- 3 tablespoons lemon juice
- 1 tablespoon caper brine
- 1 ½ teaspoon cold butter
- ⅓ cup chopped italian flat-leaf parsley, divided
- 1 ½ tablespoon cold butter
- Water, as needed

Instructions

- Heat olive oil in a heavy skillet over high heat until it just begins to smoke. Place shrimp in an even layer on the bottom of the pan and cook for 1 minute without stirring.
- Season shrimp with salt; cook and stir until shrimp begin to turn pink about 1 minute.
- Stir in garlic and red pepper flakes; cook and stir for 1 minute. Stir in lemon juice, caper brine, 1 1/2 teaspoon cold butter, and half the parsley.
- Cook until the butter has melted, about 1 minute, then turn heat to low and stir in 1 1/2 tablespoon cold butter. Cook and stir until all butter has melted to form a thick sauce and shrimp are pink and opaque about 2 to 3 minutes.
- Remove shrimp with a slotted spoon and transfer to a bowl; continue

to cook butter sauce, adding water 1 teaspoon at a time if too thick, about 2 minutes. Season with salt to taste.
- Serve shrimp topped with the pan sauce. Garnish with remaining flat-leaf parsley.

Nutrition Facts

- Calories: 196; Protein 19.1g; Carbohydrates 2.9g; Fat 12g; Cholesterol 188.1mg; Sodium 243.7mg.

26. <u>Baked Haddock</u>

Prep Time: 10 mins

Cook Time: 15 mins

Total Time: 25 mins

Servings: 4

Ingredient

- ¾ cup milk
- 2 teaspoons salt
- ¾ cup bread crumbs
- ¼ cup grated Parmesan cheese
- ¼ teaspoon ground dried thyme
- 4 haddock fillets
- ¼ cup butter, melted

Instructions

- Preheat oven to 500 degrees F (260 degrees C).
- In a small bowl, combine the milk and salt. In a separate bowl, mix the bread crumbs, Parmesan cheese, and thyme. Dip the haddock fillets in the milk, then press into the crumb mixture to coat. Place haddock fillets in a glass baking dish, and drizzle with melted butter.
- Bake on the top rack of the preheated oven until the fish flakes easily, about 15 minutes.

Nutrition Facts

- Calories: 325; Protein 27.7g; Carbohydrates 17g; Fat 15.7g; Cholesterol 103.3mg; Sodium 1565.2mg.

27. <u>Pan-Seared Tilapia</u>

Prep Time: 10 mins

Cook Time: 8 mins

Total Time: 18 mins

Servings: 4

Ingredient

- 4 (4 ounce) fillets tilapia
- Salt and pepper to taste
- ½ cup all-purpose flour
- 1 tablespoon olive oil
- 2 tablespoons unsalted butter, melted

Instructions

- Rinse tilapia fillets in cold water and pat dry with paper towels. Season both sides of each fillet with salt and pepper. Place the flour in a shallow dish; gently press each fillet into the flour to coat and shake off the excess flour.
- Heat the olive oil in a skillet over medium-high heat; cook the tilapia in the hot oil until the fish flakes easily with a fork, about 4 minutes per side. Brush the melted butter onto the tilapia at the last minute before removing it from the skillet. Serve immediately.

Nutrition Facts

- Calories: 249; Protein 24.6g; Carbohydrates 11.9g; Fat 10.8g; Cholesterol 56.3mg; Sodium 50.9mg.

28.   Classic Fish And Chips

Prep Time: 10 mins

Cook Time: 25 mins

Additional Time: 10 mins

Total Time: 45 mins

Servings: 4

Ingredient

- 4 large potatoes, peeled and cut into strips
- 1 cup all-purpose flour
- 1 teaspoon baking powder
- 1 teaspoon salt
- 1 teaspoon ground black pepper
- 1 cup milk
- 1 egg
- 1-quart vegetable oil for frying
- 1 ½ pounds cod fillets

Instructions

- Place potatoes in a medium-size bowl of cold water. In a separate medium-size mixing bowl, mix flour, baking powder, salt, and pepper. Stir in the milk and egg; stir until the mixture is smooth. Let mixture stand for 20 minutes.
- Preheat the oil in a large pot or electric skillet to 350 degrees F (175 degrees C).
- Fry the potatoes in the hot oil until they are tender. Drain them on paper towels.
- Dredge the fish in the batter, one piece at a time, and place them in the hot oil. Fry until the fish is golden brown. If necessary, increase the heat to maintain the 350 degrees F (175 degrees C) temperature. Drain well on paper towels.
- Fry the potatoes again for 1 to 2 minutes for added crispness.

Nutrition Facts

- 782 Calories: 787; Protein 44.6g; Carbohydrates 91.9g; Fat 26.2g; Cholesterol 124.6mg; Sodium 860.7mg.

29. Linguine With Clam Sauce

Prep Time: 20 mins

Cook Time: 12 mins

Total Time: 32 mins

Servings: 4

Ingredient

- 2 (6.5 ounces) cans minced clams, with juice
- ¼ cup butter
- ½ cup vegetable oil
- ½ teaspoon minced garlic
- 1 tablespoon dried parsley
- Ground black pepper to taste
- ¼ tablespoon dried basil
- 1 (16 ounces) package linguini pasta

Instructions

- Bring a large pot of salted water to boil. Cook pasta according to package directions.
- Combine clams with juice, butter, oil, minced garlic, parsley, basil, and pepper in a large saucepan. Place over medium heat until boiling. Serve warm over pasta.

Nutrition Facts

Calories: 88; Protein 37.2g; Carbohydrates 84.6g; Fat 42.7g; Cholesterol 92.3mg; Sodium 189.6mg.

30. Pan Seared Salmon I

Prep Time: 10 mins

Cook Time: 10 mins

Total Time: 20 mins

Servings: 4

Ingredient

- 4 (6 ounces) fillets of salmon
- 2 tablespoons olive oil
- 2 tablespoons capers
- ⅛ teaspoon salt
- ⅛ teaspoon ground black pepper
- 4 slices lemon

Instructions

- Preheat a large heavy skillet over medium heat for 3 minutes.
- Coat salmon with olive oil. Place in skillet, and increase heat to high. Cook for 3 minutes. Sprinkle with capers, and salt and pepper. Turn salmon over, and cook for 5 minutes, or until browned. Salmon is done when it flakes easily with a fork.
- Transfer salmon to individual plates, and garnish with lemon slices.

Nutrition Facts

- Per Serving: 371 Calories; Protein 33.7g; Carbohydrates 1.7g; Fat 25.1g; Cholesterol 99.1mg; Sodium 299.8mg.

31. Easy Extremely Garlic Shrimp

Prep Time: 10 mins

Cook Time: 10 mins

Total Time: 20 mins

Servings: 4

Ingredient

- ⅓ cup butter
- 2 teaspoons minced garlic
- 1 pound large shrimp, peeled and deveined
- 3 tablespoons garlic salt, or to taste
- 3 tablespoons garlic powder, or to taste
- ½ lemon, juiced, or to taste

Instructions

- Melt butter in a large skillet over medium heat; cook and stir minced garlic until lightly browned. Add shrimp; season with garlic salt and garlic powder. Pour lemon juice over shrimp. Continue to cook and stir until shrimp are bright pink on the outside and the meat is no longer transparent in the center, 5 to 10 minutes.

Nutrition Facts

- Calories: 254; Protein 20.1g; Carbohydrates 6.9g; Fat 16.4g; Cholesterol 213.2mg; Sodium 4386.4mg.

32.   <u>Spicy Grilled Shrimp</u>

Prep Time: 15 mins

Cook Time: 6 mins

Total Time: 21 mins

Servings: 6

Ingredient

- 1 large clove garlic
- 1 teaspoon coarse salt
- ½ teaspoon cayenne pepper
- 1 teaspoon paprika
- 2 tablespoons olive oil
- 2 teaspoons lemon juice
- 2 pounds large shrimp, peeled and deveined
- 8 wedges lemon, for garnish

Instructions

- Preheat grill for medium heat.
- In a small bowl, crush the garlic with the salt. Mix in cayenne pepper and paprika, and then stir in olive oil and lemon juice to form a paste. In a large bowl, toss shrimp with garlic paste until evenly coated.
- Lightly oil grill grate. Cook shrimp for 2 to 3 minutes per side, or until opaque. Transfer to a serving dish, garnish with lemon wedges and serve.

Nutrition Facts

- Calories: 164; Protein 25.1g; Carbohydrates 2.7g; Fat 5.9g; Cholesterol 230.4mg; Sodium 585.7mg.

33. __Sheet Pan Salmon and Bell Pepper Dinner__

Prep Time: 20 mins

Cook Time: 10 mins

Total Time: 30 mins

Servings: 4

Ingredient

- 2 tablespoons olive oil
- 4 (3 ounce) fillets salmon fillets
- 2 red bell peppers, chopped
- 1 yellow bell pepper, chopped
- 1 onion, sliced

Sauce:

- 6 tablespoons lemon juice
- 3 tablespoons olive oil
- 2 tablespoons water
- 1 tablespoon maple syrup
- 5 cloves garlic
- 1 ½ teaspoons salt
- 1 ½ teaspoon red pepper flakes
- 1 teaspoon ground cumin
- ½ bunch fresh parsley, chopped
- 1 lemon, sliced

Instructions

- Preheat oven to 400 degrees F (200 degrees C). Grease a sheet pan with 2 tablespoons olive oil.
- Place salmon fillets, red and yellow bell peppers, and onion on the prepared sheet pan.
- Combine lemon juice, 3 tablespoons olive oil, water, maple syrup, garlic, salt, red pepper flakes, cumin, and parsley in a small bowl.

Drizzle 2/3 of the sauce over the ingredients on the sheet pan.

- Bake in the preheated oven until salmon is cooked through and flakes easily with a fork, 10 to 15 minutes.
- Serve with lemon slices and remaining sauce.

Nutrition Facts

- Calories: 337; Protein 18.8g; Carbohydrates 16.9g; Fat 22.9g; Cholesterol 47mg; Sodium 920.7mg.

34. **<u>Maple Sriracha Salmon</u>**

Prep Time: 30 Min

Cook Time: 15 Min

Total Time: 45 Min

Servings: 15

Ingredients

- 1 Tbsp. brown sugar
- 2 green onions, thinly sliced
- 2 Tbsp. lime juice
- 1 tsp. finely grated lime zest
- 1 Tbsp. maple syrup
- 3 lb. salmon fillet
- ½ tsp. salt
- 2 Tbsp. sriracha sauce

Directions

- Preheat your grill on setting #4. Whisk together sriracha, lime juice, maple syrup, brown sugar, lime zest, and salt. Brush over top of salmon and let stand for 20 minutes.
- Grill, covered and without turning, for 15 to 18 minutes or until grill-marked and fish flakes easily when tested with a fork. Sprinkle with green onions before serving.

Nutrition Facts

- Calories: 327; Protein 33.7g; Carbohydrates 4g; Fat 18.5g; Cholesterol 99.1mg; Sodium 810.8mg.

33. Lemon Garlic Tilapia

Prep Time: 10 mins

Cook Time: 30 mins

Total Time: 40 mins

Servings: 4

Ingredient

- 4 each tilapia fillets
- 3 tablespoons fresh lemon juice
- 1 tablespoon butter, melted
- 1 clove garlic, finely chopped
- 1 teaspoon dried parsley flakes
- 1 dash pepper to taste

Instructions

- Preheat oven to 375 degrees F (190 degrees C). Spray a baking dish with non-stick cooking spray.
- Rinse tilapia fillets under cool water, and pat dry with paper towels.
- Place fillets in baking dish. Pour lemon juice over fillets, then drizzle butter on top. Sprinkle with garlic, parsley, and pepper.
- Bake in the preheated oven until the fish is white and flakes when pulled apart with a fork, about 30 minutes.

Nutrition Facts

- calories: 142; protein 23.1g; carbohydrates 1.4g; fat 4.4g; cholesterol 49.1mg; sodium 93mg.

35. <u>Szechwan Shrimp</u>

Prep Time: 10 mins

Cook Time: 10 mins

Total Time: 20 mins

Servings: 4

Ingredient

- 4 tablespoons water
- 2 tablespoons ketchup
- 1 tablespoon soy sauce
- 2 teaspoons cornstarch
- 1 teaspoon honey
- ½ teaspoon crushed red pepper
- ¼ teaspoon ground ginger
- 1 tablespoon vegetable oil
- ¼ cup sliced green onions
- 4 cloves garlic, minced
- 12 ounces cooked shrimp, tails removed

Instructions

- In a bowl, stir together water, ketchup, soy sauce, cornstarch, honey, crushed red pepper, and ground ginger. Set aside.
- Heat oil in a large skillet over medium-high heat. Stir in green onions and garlic; cook for 30 seconds. Stir in shrimp, and toss to coat with oil. Stir in sauce. Cook and stir until sauce are bubbly and thickened.

Nutrition Facts

- Calories: 142; Protein 18.3g; Carbohydrates 6.7g; Fat 4.4g; Cholesterol 163.8mg; Sodium 499.5mg.

36. **Lemony Steamed Fish**

Prep Time: 15 mins

Cook Time: 30 mins

Total Time: 45 mins

Servings: 6

Ingredient

- 6 (6 ounces) halibut fillets
- 1 tablespoon dried dill weed
- 1 tablespoon onion powder
- 2 teaspoons dried parsley
- ¼ teaspoon paprika
- 1 pinch seasoned salt, or more to taste
- 1 pinch lemon pepper
- 1 pinch garlic powder
- 2 tablespoons lemon juice

Instructions

- Preheat oven to 375 degrees F (190 degrees C).
- Cut 6 foil squares large enough for each fillet.
- Center fillets on the foil squares and sprinkle each with dill weed, onion powder, parsley, paprika, seasoned salt, lemon pepper, and garlic powder. Sprinkle lemon juice over each fillet. Fold foil over fillets to make a pocket and fold the edges to seal. Place sealed packets on a baking sheet.
- Bake in the preheated oven until fish flakes easily with a fork, about 30 minutes.

Nutrition Facts

- Calories: 142; protein 29.7g; carbohydrates 1.9g; fat 1.1g; cholesterol 60.7mg; sodium 183.9mg.

37. **Salmon With Fruit Salsa**

Prep Time: 15 mins Cook Time: 40 mins Total Time: 55 mins

Servings: 4

Ingredient

- 1 pound salmon steaks
- 1 lemon, juiced
- 1 tablespoon chopped fresh rosemary
- Salt and pepper to taste
- 1 lemon, sliced
- ⅓ cup water
- ¼ cup diced fresh pineapple
- ¼ cup minced onion
- 3 cloves garlic, minced
- 2 fresh jalapeno peppers, diced
- 1 tomato, diced
- ½ cup pineapple juice
- ¼ cup diced red bell pepper
- ¼ cup diced yellow bell pepper

Instructions

- Preheat oven to 350 degrees F (175 degrees C).
- Arrange salmon steaks in a shallow baking dish, and coat with lemon juice. Season with rosemary, salt, and pepper. Top with lemon slices. Pour water into the dish.
- Bake for 30 to 40 minutes in the preheated oven, or until easily flaked with a fork.
- In a medium bowl, mix pineapple, onion, garlic, jalapeno, tomato, pineapple juice, red bell pepper, and yellow bell pepper. Cover, and refrigerate while fish is baking. Top fish with salsa to serve.

Nutritional Value

- Calories: 217; Protein 25.9g; Carbohydrates 15.7g; Fat 7g; Cholesterol 50.4mg; Sodium 198.3mg.

38. Mainely Fish

Prep Time: 30 mins Cook Time: 20 mins Total Time: 50 mins Servings: 6

Ingredient

- 6 (3 ounce) fillets haddock
- salt and pepper to taste
- 4 Roma (plum) tomatoes, thinly sliced
- 1 red bell pepper, thinly sliced
- 1 yellow bell pepper, thinly sliced
- 1 small onion, thinly sliced
- 5 tablespoons capers
- 8 tablespoons chopped fresh parsley
- 6 tablespoons fresh lemon juice
- 6 tablespoons extra virgin olive oil

Instructions

- Preheat oven to 400 degrees F (200 degrees C).
- Center each piece of fish on an individual piece of aluminum foil (large enough to enclose the fish when folded). Sprinkle each piece of fish with salt and pepper. Divide the sliced tomatoes, onion, and red and yellow peppers between the 6 pieces of fish, and place them on top of the fillets. Sprinkle evenly with the capers and parsley. Drizzle each fillet with 1 tablespoon of olive oil and 1 tablespoon of lemon juice.
- Fold and seal the foil into a packet and place on a baking sheet. Leave 2 inches between each packet for even cooking.
- Bake in preheated oven for 20 minutes.
- Let rest for 5 minutes and unwrap. One packet per person.

Nutrition Facts

- Calories;: 226 Protein 17.3g; Carbohydrates 7.1g; Fat 14.4g; Cholesterol 48.4mg; Sodium 276.9mg.

39. Grilled Tuna Teriyaki

Prep Time: 15 mins

Cook Time: 10 mins

Additional Time: 30 mins

Total Time: 55 mins

Servings: 4

Ingredient

- 2 tablespoons light soy sauce
- 1 tablespoon Chinese rice wine
- 1 tablespoon minced fresh ginger root
- 1 large clove garlic, minced
- 4 (6 ounces) tuna steaks (about 3/4 inch thick)
- 1 tablespoon vegetable oil

Instructions

- Stir soy sauce, rice wine, ginger, and garlic together in a shallow dish. Place tuna in the marinade, and turn to coat. Cover the dish and refrigerate for at least 30 minutes.
- Preheat grill for medium-high heat.
- Remove tuna from marinade and discard remaining liquid. Brush both sides of steaks with oil.
- Cook tuna on the preheated grill until cooked through, 3 to 6 minutes per side.

Nutrition Facts

- Calories: 227; Protein 40.4g; Carbohydrates 1.5g; Fat 5.1g; Cholesterol 77.1mg; Sodium 328.6mg.

40. <u>Anaheim Fish Tacos</u>

Prep Time: 15 mins

Cook Time: 30 mins

Total Time: 45 mins

Servings: 6

Ingredient

- 1 teaspoon vegetable oil
- 1 anaheim chile pepper, chopped
- 1 leek, chopped
- 2 cloves garlic, crushed
- Salt and pepper to taste
- 1 cup chicken broth
- 2 large tomatoes, diced
- ½ teaspoon ground cumin
- 1 ½ pound halibut fillets
- 1 lime
- 12 corn tortillas

Instructions

- Heat the oil in a large skillet over medium heat, and saute the chile, leek, and garlic until tender and lightly browned. Season with salt and pepper.
- Mix the chicken broth and tomatoes into the skillet, and season with cumin. Bring to a boil. Reduce heat to low. Place the halibut into the mixture. Sprinkle with lime juice. Cook 15 to 20 minutes until the halibut is easily flaked with a fork. Wrap in warmed corn tortillas to serve.

Nutrition Facts

- Calories: 273; Protein 27.7g; Carbohydrates 29.9g; Fat 5.1g; Cholesterol 36.3mg; Sodium 285.8mg.

41. <u>**Batter Fried Basa Fish**</u>

Prep Time: 15 mins

Cook Time: 20 mins

Total Time: 35 mins

Ingredients

- Boneless Basa fillet – 2
- All-purpose flour (Maida) – 1 cup
- Egg – 2
- Milk – 1 cup
- Salt to taste
- Vegetable oil – 1 tsp + more for shallow frying
- Freshly crushed black pepper – ½ tsp or more as per taste

Instructions

- Wash the fish fillet well. I used frozen fillets, so I had to thaw them completely before starting. Season the fillet with a pinch of salt on both sides.
- In a big bowl, combine the flour, eggs, milk, salt [approximately a little less than ½ teaspoon will do], and 1 teaspoon of oil.
- Whisk them well to make a thick and smooth batter. The batter must be very smooth without any lumps. Consistency should be such that it should adhere to the fish fillet covering all sides and does not drip off completely. [See notes below for more details.]
- Heat oil in a non-stick frying pan. I didn't deep fry my fish; I did shallow frying which worked quite well.
- Dip a fillet into the batter. Take it out, let the excess batter drip off and when the oil is quite hot, tip in the batter-coated fish on the pan. If you find that the batter is flowing out of the fillet, take a little amount of batter from the bowl using a spoon and smear it on the top of the fillet. Do not move the fish for 2 minutes and let it cook on medium-low flame.
- When the bottom side of the fillet turns golden brown after about 5 minutes on medium flame, carefully flip the fillet and fry the other

side till it turns golden brown. It will take around 5 to 6 minutes on each side but it also depends on the thickness of the fillets you are using. Mine took about 6 minutes on each side. To check the doneness, take a toothpick and prick the fish in the middle. If it goes in very easily without any resistance, your fish is done. Else give it two more minutes.

- Once done, take out the batter-fried basa fillets on a plate lined with an absorbent kitchen towel to soak the excess oil.
- Serve the batter-fried basa warm with tartar sauce on the side. Enjoy!

Nutrition Facts

- Calories: 142; Protein 18.3g; Carbohydrates 6.7g; Fat 4.4g; Cholesterol 163.8mg; Sodium 499.5mg.

42. Lemon-Garlic Marinated Shrimp

Total Time: 10 mins

Servings: 12

Ingredient

- 3 tablespoons minced garlic
- 2 tablespoons extra-virgin olive oil
- ¼ cup lemon juice
- ¼ cup minced fresh parsley
- ½ teaspoon kosher salt
- ½ teaspoon pepper
- 1 ¼ pounds cooked shrimp

Instructions

Place garlic and oil in a small skillet and cook over medium heat until fragrant, about 1 minute. Add lemon juice, parsley, salt, and pepper. Toss with shrimp in a large bowl. Chill until ready to serve.

Nutrition Facts

- Calories: 82; Protein 11g; Carbohydrates 1.9g; Dietary Fiber 0.1g; Sugars 0.2g; Fat 3.2g;; Calcium 49.3mg; Iron 0.3mg; Magnesium 19.1mg; Potassium 102.3mg; Sodium 495.3mg.

43. Shrimp Poke

Active Time: 30 mins Total Time: 30 mins Servings: 4

Ingredient

- ¾ cup thinly sliced scallion greens
- ¼ cup reduced-sodium tamari
- 1 ½ tablespoons mirin
- 1 ½ tablespoon toasted (dark) sesame oil
- 1 tablespoon white sesame seeds
- 2 teaspoons grated fresh ginger
- ½ teaspoon crushed red pepper (Optional)
- 12 ounces cooked shrimp, cut into 1/2-inch pieces
- 2 cups cooked brown rice
- 2 tablespoons rice vinegar
- 2 cups sliced cherry tomatoes
- 2 cups diced avocado
- ¼ cup chopped cilantro
- ¼ cup toasted black sesame seeds

Instructions

- Whisk scallion greens, tamari, mirin, oil, white sesame seeds, ginger, and crushed red pepper, if using, in a medium bowl. Set aside 2 tablespoons of the sauce in a small bowl. Add shrimp to the sauce in the medium bowl and gently toss to coat.
- Combine rice and vinegar in a large bowl. Divide among 4 bowls and top each with 3/4 cup shrimp, 1/2 cup each tomato and avocado, and 1 tablespoon each cilantro and black sesame seeds. Drizzle with the reserved sauce and serve.

Nutrition Facts

- Calories: 460; Protein 28.9g; Carbohydrates 40.2g; Dietary Fiber 9.9g; Sugars 4.5g; Fat 22.1g; Saturated Fat 3.2g;; Calcium 113.2mg; Iron 3.2mg; Magnesium 145.1mg; Potassium 939.3mg; Sodium 860.6mg.

44. Creamy Lemon Pasta With Shrimp

Active Time: 20 mins

Total Time: 20 mins

Servings: 4

Ingredients

- 8 ounces whole-wheat fettuccine
- 1 tablespoon extra-virgin olive oil
- 12 ounces sustainably sourced peeled and deveined raw shrimp (26-30 per pound)
- 2 tablespoons unsalted butter
- 1 tablespoon finely chopped garlic
- ¼ teaspoon crushed red pepper
- 4 cups loosely packed arugula
- ¼ cup whole-milk plain yogurt
- 1 teaspoon lemon zest
- 2 tablespoons lemon juice
- ¼ teaspoon salt
- ⅓ cup grated Parmesan cheese, plus more for garnish
- ¼ cup thinly sliced fresh basil

Instructions

- Bring 7 cups of water to a boil. Add fettuccine, stirring to separate the noodles. Cook until just tender, 7 to 9 minutes. Reserve 1/2 cup of the cooking water and drain.
- Meanwhile, heat oil in a large nonstick skillet over medium-high heat. Add shrimp and cook, stirring occasionally, until pink and curled, 2 to 3 minutes. Transfer the shrimp to a bowl.
- Add butter to the pan and reduce heat to medium. Add garlic and crushed red pepper; cook, stirring often, until the garlic is fragrant, about 1 minute. Add arugula and cook, stirring, until wilted, about 1 minute. Reduce heat to low. Add the fettuccine, yogurt, lemon zest, and the reserved cooking water, 1/4 cup at a time, tossing well, until the fettuccine is fully coated and creamy. Add the shrimp, lemon

juice, and salt, tossing to coat the fettuccine. Remove from the heat and toss with Parmesan.

- Serve the fettuccine topped with basil and more Parmesan, if desired.

Nutrition Facts

- Calories: 403; Protein 28.3g; Carbohydrates 45.5g; Dietary Fiber 5.8g; Sugars 3g; Fat 13.9g;; Calcium 207.5mg; Iron 3mg; Magnesium 124.7mg; Potassium 626.4mg; Sodium 396.3mg.

45. <u>Grilled Blackened Shrimp Tacos</u>

Active Time: 20 mins

Total Time: 20 mins

Servings: 4

Ingredient

- 1 ripe avocado
- 1 tablespoon lime juice
- 1 small clove garlic, grated
- ¼ teaspoon salt
- 1 pound large raw shrimp (16-20 count), peeled and deveined
- 2 tablespoons salt-free Cajun spice blend
- 8 corn tortillas, warmed
- 2 cups iceberg lettuce, chopped
- ½ cup fresh cilantro leaves
- ½ cup prepared pico de gallo

Instructions

- Preheat grill to medium-high.
- Mash avocado with a fork in a small bowl. Add lime juice, garlic, and salt and stir to combine.
- Pat shrimp dry. Toss the shrimp with Cajun seasoning in a medium bowl. Thread onto four 10- to 12-inch metal skewers. Grill, turning once until the shrimp are just cooked through, about 4 minutes total.
- Serve the shrimp in tortillas, topped with guacamole, lettuce, cilantro, and pico de gallo.

Nutrition Facts

- Calories: 286; Protein 24g; Carbohydrates 30.4g; Dietary Fiber 6.9g; Sugars 3.5g; Fat 9.3g; Calcium 117.8mg; Iron 1.6mg; Magnesium 87.2mg; Potassium 662.1mg; Sodium 442.7mg;

46. Moqueca (Seafood & Coconut Chowder)

Active Time: 30 mins

Total Time: 30 mins

Servings: 8

Ingredient

- 1 pound fresh crabmeat (preferably claw meat), cleaned and picked over
- 1 pound raw shrimp (16-20 per pound), peeled and deveined if desired
- ¼ cup lemon juice
- 1 ½ tablespoons dendê (red palm oil; see Tip) or canola oil
- 3 cups sliced red bell peppers
- 2 ½ cups sliced green bell peppers
- 2 ½ cups sliced red onions
- ½ cup minced fresh cilantro, plus more for garnish
- 4 large cloves garlic, minced
- ¼ cup tomato paste
- ¾ teaspoon salt
- ¾ teaspoon ground pepper
- 2 14-ounce cans of coconut milk
- 2 cups clam juice or fish stock
- 4 cups cooked brown rice

Instructions

- Combine crab, shrimp, and lemon juice in a medium bowl.
- Heat oil in a large pot over medium-high heat. Add red peppers, green peppers, and onions; cook, stirring occasionally, until beginning to soften, about 4 minutes. Add cilantro, garlic, tomato paste, salt, and pepper; cook, stirring, for 1 minute. Add coconut milk and clam juice (or fish stock) and bring to a simmer. Reduce heat to maintain a simmer, cover, and cook until the peppers are softened, 8 to 10 minutes.
- Add the crab and shrimp and return to a simmer over medium heat.

Cover and cook until the shrimp is cooked through, 3 to 4 minutes more. Serve the chowder over rice. Garnish with cilantro, if desired.

Nutrition Facts

- Calories: 485 Fat 26g; Cholesterol 112mg; Sodium 686mg; Carbohydrates 39g; Dietary Fiber 5g; Protein 28g; Sugars 5g; Saturated Fat 20g.

47. __Brodetto Di Pesce (Adriatic-Style Seafood Stew)__

Active Time: 45 mins

Total Time: 1 hr 15 mins

Servings: 8

Ingredient

- ¼ Cup extra-virgin olive oil, plus more for serving
- 1 medium yellow or red onion, finely diced
- ⅓ cup finely diced celery
- ⅓ cup finely chopped flat-leaf parsley, plus more for serving
- 4 cloves garlic, lightly crushed, divided
- ½ teaspoon crushed red pepper
- ¾ cup dry white wine
- 3 sprigs of fresh oregano
- 3 fresh bay leaves
- 2 1/2 cups clam juice or seafood stock, divided
- 2 cups petite diced or crushed canned tomatoes
- 2 pounds littleneck clams, scrubbed
- 1 pound mussels, scrubbed
- 1 pound cleaned squid tubes or tentacles, tubes cut into rings
- 1 pound meaty white fish, such as cod, monkfish, rockfish, snapper, or a combination, cut into 2-inch pieces
- 2 tablespoons lemon juice
- 8 diagonal slices whole-grain baguette (1/2 inch thick), plus more for serving

Instructions

- Cook oil, onion, celery, parsley, 3 cloves garlic, and crushed red pepper in a large pot over medium-low heat, stirring occasionally, until the vegetables are very tender, about 15 minutes.
- Increase heat to medium-high and add wine; cook for 1 minute. Add oregano and bay leaves; cook for 30 seconds. Add 2 cups clam juice

(or stock) and tomatoes and bring to a boil over high heat. Reduce heat to a simmer and cook until slightly thickened, 20 to 25 minutes.

- Add clams and mussels; cover and cook for 5 minutes. Add squid, fish, and the remaining 1/2 cup clam juice (or stock). Cover and cook until the fish is just cooked through, 8 to 12 minutes. Remove from heat and gently stir in lemon juice.
- Meanwhile, preheat the broiler to high.
- Place bread on a rimmed baking sheet and broil until lightly browned for 1 to 2 minutes. Immediately rub with the remaining garlic clove.
- Place one slice of bread in each of 8 shallow bowls and top with the stew. Serve with more oil, parsley, and bread, if desired.

Nutrition Facts

- Calories: 334; Protein 31g; Carbohydrates 25.7g; Dietary Fiber 2.1g; Sugars 4.2g; Fat 10.2g; Saturated Fat 1.5g; Calcium 97.2mg; Iron 5.3mg; Magnesium 77.1mg; Potassium 902.6mg; Sodium 770.3mg.

48. <u>Seafood Linguine</u>

Total Time: 35 mins

Servings: 4

Ingredient

- 8 ounces whole-wheat linguine, or spaghetti
- 2 tablespoons extra-virgin olive oil
- 4 cloves garlic, chopped
- 1 tablespoon chopped shallot
- 1 28-ounce can diced tomatoes, drained
- ½ cup white wine
- ½ teaspoon salt
- ¼ teaspoon freshly ground pepper
- 12 littleneck or small cherrystone clams, (about 1 pound), scrubbed
- 8 ounces dry sea scallops
- 8 ounces tilapia, or other flaky white fish, cut into 1-inch strips
- 1 tablespoon chopped fresh marjoram or 1 teaspoon dried, plus more for garnish
- 1/4 cup grated Parmesan cheese, (optional)

Instructions

- Bring a large pot of water to a boil. Add pasta and cook until just tender, 8 to 10 minutes, or according to package directions. Drain and rinse.
- Meanwhile, heat oil in a large skillet over medium heat. Add garlic and shallot and cook, stirring, until beginning to soften, about 1 minute.
- Increase the heat to medium-high. Add tomatoes, wine, salt, and pepper. Bring to a simmer and cook for 1 minute. Add clams, cover, and cook for 2 minutes. Stir in scallops, fish, and marjoram. Cover and cook until the scallops and fish are cooked through and the clams have opened, 3 to 5 minutes more. (Discard any clams that don't open.)
- Spoon the sauce and clams over the pasta and sprinkle with additional marjoram and Parmesan (if using).

Nutrition Facts

- Calories: 460; Protein 34.5g; Carbohydrates 55.8g; Dietary Fiber 8.2g; Sugars 7.5g; Fat 9.5g; Saturated Fat 1.6g; Calcium 86.5mg; Iron 4.5mg; Magnesium 122.1mg; Potassium 474.9mg; Sodium 1173.3mg.

49. __Seafood Paella With Spring Vegetables__

Active Time: 1 hr 15 mins

Total Time: 1 hr 35 mins

Servings: 6

Ingredient

- 6 tablespoons extra-virgin olive oil, divided
- 2 cups diced onion
- 1 cup diced fennel
- 3 medium tomatoes, grated on the large holes of a box grater (skins discarded)
- 4 cloves garlic, thinly sliced
- 2 tablespoons white-wine vinegar
- 1 teaspoon sea salt, divided
- ½ teaspoon ground pepper
- ½ teaspoon crushed red pepper
- Pinch of saffron
- 1 large fresh artichoke
- 1 cup Calasparra rice or other paella rice
- 2 cups seafood stock
- 1 cup green beans, trimmed and cut into 2-inch pieces
- 4 ounces squid bodies, sliced into rings
- 6-12 clams and/or mussels, scrubbed
- 8 ounces skinned monkfish or cod, cut into 1-inch-thick pieces

Instructions

- Heat 3 tablespoons oil in a 13- to 14-inch paella pan over medium-high heat. Add onion and fennel; cook, stirring often, until the onion is translucent, about 5 minutes. Add tomatoes, garlic, vinegar, 1/2 teaspoon salt, pepper, crushed red pepper, and saffron. Reduce heat to maintain a simmer and cook, stirring occasionally, until the tomato liquid has evaporated, 20 to 25 minutes.
- Meanwhile, clean artichoke. Cut lengthwise into 6 wedges. Heat 2 tablespoons oil in a large skillet over medium heat until very hot but

not smoking. Add the artichoke wedges; sprinkle with 1/8 teaspoon salt and cook until browned, about 2 minutes per side. Transfer to a plate.

- Preheat oven to 375 degrees F.
- When the tomato liquid has evaporated, add rice to the paella pan, increase heat to medium, and cook, stirring, for 2 minutes. Add stock. Turn on a second burner so both the front and rear burner on one side of the stove are on; bring to a boil over high heat.
- Spread the rice evenly in the pan and nestle the artichokes and beans into it. Reduce heat to maintain a low simmer and cook for 10 minutes, rotating and shifting the pan around the burners periodically to help the rice cook evenly. Season squid with 1/8 teaspoon salt and place on the rice. Cook, without stirring but continuing to rotate the pan, for 5 minutes more.
- Nestle clams and/or mussels into the rice with the open edges facing up. Season fish with the remaining 1/4 teaspoon salt and place on top of the rice. Remove the paella from the heat and very carefully cover the pan with foil.
- Transfer the pan to the oven and bake for 10 minutes. Let stand, covered, for 10 minutes before serving.

To Prep A Fresh Artichoke:

1. Trim 1/2 to 1 inch from the stem end. Peel the stem with a vegetable peeler.

2. Trim 1/2 inch off the top.

3. Remove the small, tough outer leaves from the stem end and snip all spiky tips from the remaining outer leaves using kitchen shears.

4. Cut in half lengthwise and scoop out the fuzzy choke with a melon baller or grapefruit spoon.

Keep artichokes from browning by rubbing the cut edges with a lemon half or putting them in a large bowl of ice water with lemon juice.

Nutrition Facts

354 calories; protein 16.1g; carbohydrates 38.2g; dietary fiber 4.7g; sugars 5.2g; fat 15.3g; saturated fat 2.3g; calcium 65.6mg; iron 1.7mg; magnesium 51.4mg; potassium 695.1mg; sodium 695.3mg;

50. <u>Spaghetti With Garlic & Clam Sauce</u>

Total Time: 45 mins

Servings: 8

Ingredient

- 2 heads garlic
- 28 fresh littleneck clams, scrubbed and rinsed well
- ¾ cup cold water
- 5 tablespoons extra-virgin olive oil, divided
- 2 tablespoons all-purpose flour
- 1 cup dry white wine, such as Pinot Grigio
- 1 cup chopped fresh parsley plus 2 tablespoons, divided
- 1 tablespoon chopped fresh tarragon
- ¾ teaspoon freshly ground pepper, divided
- 1/8 teaspoon crushed red pepper (optional)
- 1 pound whole-wheat spaghetti or linguine

Instructions

- Put a large pot of water on to boil.
- Peel 1 head of garlic, separate cloves, and halve any large ones. Peel the second head and chop all the cloves.
- Place clams in a Dutch oven or large saucepan with cold water. Cover and cook over high heat, stirring frequently, until the shells just open, 6 to 10 minutes. Transfer to a bowl as they open, making sure to keep all the juice in the pan. Discard any unopened clams. Reserve 16 whole clams in their shells. Then, working over the pot so you don't lose any of the juice, remove the meat from the remaining clams. Coarsely chop the meat; set aside separately from the whole clams. Pour the clam juice from the pan into a medium bowl, being careful not to include any of the sediment. Rinse and dry the pan.
- Heat 4 tablespoons of oil in the pan over medium heat. Add all the garlic and cook, stirring, for 1 minute. Stir in the chopped clams and cook for 15 seconds. Add flour and cook, stirring, for 15 seconds. Increase heat to high, stir in wine and the reserved clam juice. Bring the sauce to a simmer, stirring constantly to prevent the flour from

clumping. Once it's simmering, reduce the heat to medium and stir in 1 cup parsley, tarragon, and 1/2 teaspoon pepper. Cook, stirring often, until slightly thickened, 6 to 8 minutes. Add crushed red pepper, if using. Add the reserved clams in shells and stir to coat with the sauce.

- Meanwhile, cook pasta in boiling water until al dente, 10 to 13 minutes, or according to package directions. Stir 2 tablespoons of the pasta-cooking water into the clam sauce, then drain the pasta and transfer to a large serving dish. Stir the remaining 1 tablespoon oil and 1/4 teaspoon pepper into the pasta. Spoon the clams and sauce over the pasta. Sprinkle with the remaining 2 tablespoons parsley.

Nutrition Facts

- Calories: 371; Protein 17.8g; Carbohydrates 49.6g; Dietary Fiber 7.3g; Sugars 2.5g; Fat 10.3g; Saturated Fat 1.5g;; Calcium 83mg; Iron 3.8mg; Magnesium 97mg; Potassium 431.8mg; Sodium 412mg;

CPSIA information can be obtained
at www.ICGtesting.com
Printed in the USA
LVHW050753040621
689237LV00006B/383